Ulvan Ozad

Cartilage Regeneration

AF153279

Ulvan Ozad

Cartilage Regeneration

LAP LAMBERT Academic Publishing

Impressum / Imprint

Bibliografische Information der Deutschen Nationalbibliothek: Die Deutsche Nationalbibliothek verzeichnet diese Publikation in der Deutschen Nationalbibliografie; detaillierte bibliografische Daten sind im Internet über http://dnb.d-nb.de abrufbar.

Alle in diesem Buch genannten Marken und Produktnamen unterliegen warenzeichen-, marken- oder patentrechtlichem Schutz bzw. sind Warenzeichen oder eingetragene Warenzeichen der jeweiligen Inhaber. Die Wiedergabe von Marken, Produktnamen, Gebrauchsnamen, Handelsnamen, Warenbezeichnungen u.s.w. in diesem Werk berechtigt auch ohne besondere Kennzeichnung nicht zu der Annahme, dass solche Namen im Sinne der Warenzeichen- und Markenschutzgesetzgebung als frei zu betrachten wären und daher von jedermann benutzt werden dürften.

Bibliographic information published by the Deutsche Nationalbibliothek: The Deutsche Nationalbibliothek lists this publication in the Deutsche Nationalbibliografie; detailed bibliographic data are available in the Internet at http://dnb.d-nb.de.

Any brand names and product names mentioned in this book are subject to trademark, brand or patent protection and are trademarks or registered trademarks of their respective holders. The use of brand names, product names, common names, trade names, product descriptions etc. even without a particular marking in this work is in no way to be construed to mean that such names may be regarded as unrestricted in respect of trademark and brand protection legislation and could thus be used by anyone.

Coverbild / Cover image: www.ingimage.com

Verlag / Publisher:
LAP LAMBERT Academic Publishing
ist ein Imprint der / is a trademark of
OmniScriptum GmbH & Co. KG
Heinrich-Böcking-Str. 6-8, 66121 Saarbrücken, Deutschland / Germany
Email: info@lap-publishing.com

Herstellung: siehe letzte Seite /
Printed at: see last page
ISBN: 978-3-659-63904-3

Zugl. / Approved by: Barts and the London, Queen Mary University of London, Diss., 2014

Table of Contents

To my biggest wish in life, Murat...

Introduction

Growing chondrocytes artificially into a morphology resembling real life or repairing a degenerated cartilage tissue is very challenging. Articular cartilage present in joints is not homogenous; various arrangement of chondrocytes with different morphologies and matrix compositions are present in different zones. Moreover, lack of vascular supply to chondrocytes creates difficulties for cartilage repair and regeneration.

Arthritis is a very common condition creating disability within the population. Osteoarthritis and rheumatoid arthritis are the most common types of arthritis causing degenerative changes in the joints, pain and loss of movement in the joint.

There is no definitive treatment for arthritis and long term management eventually resulting in disability and pain creates a burden not only on the patient, but also on the society and the health system.

All treatment modalities currently present in the field aim to temporarily manage the condition and prevent progression. Both osteoarthritis and rheumatoid arthritis involve components of inflammation resulting in cartilage destruction. However the components, pathways and suppression of inflammatory reactions is very complex and is still being researched.

Understanding the pro-inflammatory and anti-inflammatory reactions within cartilage along with signalling pathways would enable to seek a treatment for these conditions through suppressing the inflammatory reactions or promoting the anti-inflammatory reactions.

Current methods for managing arthritis in joints involve NSAIDs, corticosteroids and biological agents which aim to manage the intracellular disintegration; and, surgical methods such as debridement, marrow stimulation, autologous chondrocyte implantation and osteochondral transplantation that aim to either promote new tissue formation or replacement of damaged tissue with healthy cartilage. None of the current treatments create a solution for cartilage repair or regeneration.

New therapeutic innovations are required for permanent treatment of cartilage damage; and, the most promising pathway to this is through modulation and prevention of the inflammatory pathway in disease process.

Chondrocyte repair is one of the most challenging processes which is still not clearly acknowledged in the regenerative medicine field. Understanding numerous factors such as the structure and function of cartilage, common damage processes such as osteoarthritis and rheumatoid arthritis, inflammatory process pathway within the joint, current problems in cartilage regeneration, available cartilage repair methods and impact of this problem on public would assist finding a sustainable permanent solution to this problem.

Structure and Function of Cartilage

There are three types of cartilage in humans with different structures and functions; elastic cartilage, fibrocartilage and hyaline cartilage. All three cartilage types have a varying collagen and proteoglycan content as well as different chondrocyte morphologies. Elastic cartilage is abundant in the regions that require strength as the elastic fibres present in cartilage facilitate the stretching process. Fibrocartilage, on the other hand, is present in regions where pressure is applied on such as intervertebral discs (Tortora and Derrickson, 2006). Hyaline cartilage is the most abundant cartilage type present in the body and is surrounded by the perichondrium. Large quantity of collagen fibres are present in hyaline cartilage compared to the small chondrocyte quantity (Marieb and Hoehn, 2009).

Structure of hyaline cartilage is clinically very important as hyaline cartilage is present in the joints and acts as a compression absorber at the articular cartilage in the joints. There are four articular cartilage layers with different cell morphologies and matrix contents. The superficial layer (tangential layer) has flat chondrocytes, very high collagen content which is aligned as fibres parallel to surface and a little amount of proteoglycan.

Transitional layer (intermediate layer), which is the middle zone, has spherical chondrocytes. In this layer, collagen fibres are randomly aligned and is abundant of proteoglycans.

Deep zone named as the radial layer has parallel arrangement of chondrocytes and collagen fibres are aligned perpendicular to the surface. In this layer, small number of chondrocytes exist together in columns named as lacunae.

Calcified cartilage layer is the deepest zone present in articular cartilage and it separates hyaline cartilage from the subchondral bone (Wheeless, 2011).

Chondrocytes are heterogeneously distributed throughout different zones of the cartilage (Hall, 1998). Their main purpose is production and maintenance of extracellular matrix. Chondrocytes exist in functional units named as chondrons. In chondrons, several chondrocytes are surrounded by a matrix rich in proteoglycans and negligible amounts of collagen (Poole et al., 1992).

Chondrocytic lineage follows the pathway of colony forming unit-fibroblast, mesenchymal stem cell, chondrocyte and hypertrophic chondrocyte. Mesenchymal stem cells differentiate into various osteochondrogenic cells and these cells then differentiate into chondroblasts which facilitate the synthesis of extracellular matrix (ECM). Entrapment of chondroblasts in lacunae disconnects the cell from the ECM and converts it into a chondrocyte (Lee et al., 2013).

Chondrocytes are the mature cells found in cartilage. These cells are present as groups in lacunae; and, because of the rigid construction of cartilage, cells could not spread out. Depending on the location, chondrocyte reproduction is very restricted.

Interstitial cartilage growth takes place by division of chondrocytes and production of ECM which causes scattering of chondrocytes resulting in an expansion in size of the cartilage. Appositional growth primarily takes place due to division and differentiation of fibroblasts into chondroblasts (Tortora and Derrickson, 2006).

Chondroblasts are the cells found in growing areas of cartilage. These cells secrete matrix including type 2 collagen and the ground substance which is made up of collagen and proteoglycans (Blitterswijk et al., 2005).

There is no blood and nervous supply to chondrocytes. Nutrients are received and waste removal is achieved by diffusion from perichondrium. This is the key reason behind the slow growth and repair of chondrocytes. Due to superficial zone and deep calcified zone being anatomically closer to the blood supply, proliferation primarily happens in these zones (Blitterswijk et al., 2005).

Chondrocytes are primarily anaerobic; therefore, glucose is very important for the survival of chondrocytes. In the absence of glucose, chondrocytes perform oxidative respiration and oxygen becomes important in these situations (Heywood, 2006).

ECM is very important for an effectively functioning cartilage and play a great role in regulation of mechanical cartilage characteristics. ECM synthesis is performed by chondrocytes and mechanical loading is key in production and maintenance (Grodzinsky et al., 2000). The conversion pathway of the mechanical stimuli into a biological response inside chondrocytes has not been clearly understood yet.

The majority of ECM is made up of water (Marieb and Hoehn, 2009). Ability of the tissue fluid to move because of the water content not only protects the chondrocytes by rebounding if there is compression, but also helps for nourishment of chondrocytes. Resistance to any applied force on cartilage is accomplished by type 2 collagen present in ECM. Proteoglycans present in the extracellular matrix is important for facilitation of solute flow (Kuhnel et al., 2003).

A biphasic system is created in cartilage by the ionic water content of chondrocytes and extracellular matrix (Mow and Wang, 1999). Proteoglycans which are negatively charged bind to the positive ions present in the water; and, total charge in the system directs the flow of water. Negative charge causes water inflow until an equilibrium point is reached where pressure due to inflow and stress on matrix caused by compressive forces are equal (Cohen et al., 1998). High compressive force or hydrodynamic inflow results in non-achievement of this equilibrium and could cause a damage on chondrocytes.

Although immature articular cartilage has the ability to recover and repair, mature cartilage could not heal spontaneously (Hunter, 1747; Namba et al., 1998). The reason for this could be due to several differences between immature and mature cartilage tissue.

Immature chondrocytes have a higher cell density, higher messenger RNA levels and better ECM production rate compared to mature adult cartilage (Stockwell and Meachim, 1979). Lack of vascularisation and high density of the matrix content lead to immune deficiencies in the articular cartilage (Gibson et al., 1958; Gross et al., 2008).

Chondrocyte cell division which is normally very restricted, declines even more with increasing age; and, the damage created on cartilage stays permanent in human body causing pain and limitation in joint movement.

Trauma, degenerative conditions or inflammation can cause damage to cartilage. High lifespan in developing countries resulting in increased body degeneration cause degenerative joint diseases affecting cartilage such as osteoarthritis. Moreover, autoimmune and inflammatory reactions in body could cause arthritis. On average, 20 million arthritis, 20 million cartilage defect and one million knee trauma patients are treated every year (Husing et al., 2003). Understanding the pathophysiology, manifestations and management of these conditions is essential for achieving chondrocyte repair.

Osteoarthritis

Osteoarthritis is the most common arthritic condition in the United Kingdom (Osteoarthritis, 2012). Prevalence is significantly higher in older people. Osteoarthritis mainly takes place in weight-bearing joints and it could be caused by mechanical factors such as trauma or excessive use of joints as well as old age, obesity or hereditary conditions.

Osteoarthritis mainly affects the weight bearing joints which are knees and hips but it can also occur in hands and spine. Articular cartilage in weight bearing joints is exposed to friction due to movement and compressive force causing defects and lesions in the cartilage (NHS Choices, 2009). It results in inflammation of the joint space, restricted range of joint movement, muscle weakness around the joint, joint destruction and osteophyte (new bone spurs) formation.

Main symptoms of osteoarthritis are pain, loss in range of movement and joint stiffness. Bony enlargements in distal interphalangeal joints (Herbeden's nodes) and proximal interphalangeal joints (Bouchard's nodes) are characteristics of osteoarthritis in hands. On radiograph of an osteoarthritic joint, narrow joint space is observed as well as cyst formation in subchondral bone, sclerotic lesions and osteophytes.

Injury to cartilage could happen either as partial or full thickness, affecting cartilage and the subchondral bone. Partial thickness injuries are superficial whereas full thickness injuries happen in chondral and subchondral layers, repaired by filling of the fibrocollagenous tissue.

As blood supply is absent to cartilage, drilling, microfractures or operations such as arthroplasty could increase the formation of fibrocollagenous tissue resulting in premature osteoarthritis (Buckwalter and Mankin, 1998).

In physiologically normal cartilage, type 2 collagen is the collagen type abundant; however, collagen type 1 is produced more in osteoarthritis and this affects stability of the matrix. Decreased aggrecan content of ECM can be detected in osteoarthritis. Reduced proteoglycan content exposes the cartilage to more damage caused by loading.

There is no definitive treatment for osteoarthritis. Management aims to reduce the rate of degeneration and prevent pain as much as possible. Exercise, weight loss, painkillers, anti-inflammatory medications and joint replacement surgery are used in temporary management of the condition (Colledge et al., 2010).

Primary cause of osteoarthritis is abnormal loading on joint or inability to repair the defect. Secondary osteoarthritis is caused by other factors such as diabetes, Marfan syndrome and Ehlers-Danlos syndrome.

Ageing is important in progression of osteoarthritis because as the proteoglycan content decreases, water content of joints also decrease by increasing age. This results in cartilage being not resilient. When proteoglycan content is reduced, collagen becomes more susceptible to degeneration. Mild inflammation in pericapsullar area also takes place due to the breakdown products from the cartilage damage.

The first step of osteoarthritis management is lifestyle modification. Weight loss is very important since it decreases the amount of applied force and stress on the joint. Low intensity physical exercise is also advised as a lifestyle modification.

Medical treatment involves analgesic and anti-inflammatory medications to relieve the pain and supress the inflammation caused by degradation products. Paracetamol and non-steroidal anti-inflammatory drugs (NSAIDs) are the main drug treatments for osteoarthritis. Local glucocorticoid injections like hydrocortisone was also found to provide short term pain relief (Arroll et al., 2004).

The final choice of management is joint replacement surgery. Prosthetic joints function successfully in the body up to a maximum of 15 years and early insertion of prostheses would require revision surgery; there is infection and failure risk in the operation as well; therefore, joint replacement surgery is considered when all other treatment modalities are exhausted.

Rheumatoid Arthritis

Rheumatoid arthritis is a common systemic inflammatory process which frequently affects the middle aged people. In arthritis, synovial membrane is inflamed. It most commonly happens in small joints. Synovitis causes erosion on the articular cartilage which in turn limits the range of movement and causes pain.

Rheumatoid arthritis affects women three times more than men. There is symmetrical joint involvement, early morning stiffness, joint deformity, decreased range of movement as well as systemic symptoms such as fever and fatigue. (Lee and Weinblatt, 2001). Rheumatoid arthritis manifests as early morning stiffness and pain whereas in osteoarthritis, pain increases with activity.

The underlying mechanism of rheumatoid arthritis is not clearly known. There is presence of an inflammatory reaction that targets the joints as well as demonstrating systemic manifestations such as inflammatory heart conditions or rheumatoid nodules.

Rheumatoid arthritis is symmetrically distributed and most commonly affected joints are found in distal parts. The articular characteristics of rheumatoid arthritis are joint tenderness, synovial thickening, joint effusion, decreased range of motion, erythema, joint subluxation and ankylosis. It can also cause generalised systemic symptoms such as weakness, fever, weight loss, anaemia, mononeuritis and depression.

Extra-articular involvement of rheumatoid arthritis could be found on skin as rheumatoid nodules and vasculitis; in eye as keratoconjunctivitis, irisitis or episcleritis; in pulmonary system as fibrosis or effusion; in cardiac system as myocarditis; or, elsewhere in other body regions (Lee and Weinblatt, 2001).

Signs of rheumatoid arthritis in cellular level are the presence of inflammatory cells, increased amount of cytokines and formation of a granulation tissue (pannus) within the joint. As a result of these, there is destruction to the underlying cartilage.

Rheumatoid factor and anticyclic citrulinated peptide are the main antibodies found in rheumatoid arthritis. These antibodies are thought to contribute to formation of immune complexes and release of pro-inflammatory mediators (Van Venrooj et al., 2008). Tumour necrosis factor α (TNF-α) and interleukin 1β (IL 1β) are the cytokines found in high amounts in rheumatoid arthritis (Wood et al., 1992). TNF-α stimulates prostaglandin E_2 (PGE_2) and collagenase production in synovial cells (Kunisch et al., 2009) and IL1β initiates proteolysis process in rheumatoid arthritis (Wood et al., 1992).

Identifying antigens specific to diseases is important for understanding pathology. Numerous antigens have been identified in rheumatoid arthritis as high molecular weight antigens such as fibrinogen gamma chain, gelsolin, ceruloplasmin, alpha-2 macroglobulin; and, low molecular weight antigens such as amyloid, c-reactive protein, albumin, fibrinogen, C3 complement (Biswas et al., 2013).

Arthritis is a non-resolving inflammatory disorder and medications such as methotrexate and sulphasalazine could mediate the resolution of inflammation (Gilroy et al., 2004). Disease modifying anti-rheumatic drugs (DMARDs) are the primary treatment of rheumatoid arthritis. Most commonly used DMARD is methotrexate followed by sulfasalazine. Other medications such as gold and cyclosporine are used less due to their side effects.

If monotherapy does not efficiently manage the condition, combination therapy could be used as combination therapy has proven to have benefits in rheumatoid arthritis treatment (Lee and Weinblatt, 2001). DMARD therapy decreases the inflammatory markers but irreversible joint destruction continues (Mulherin et al., 1986).

If management with DMARDs does not provide any benefit to the patient for 3 months, biological agents could be used to treat rheumatoid arthritis. In TNF biological response modifiers, etanercept has an action against both TNF-α and β whereas infliximab is against only TNF-α (Lee and Weinblatt, 2001). TNF-α biological response modifiers have generated a great interest for creation of future therapies but toxicity and systemic side effects are creating a great concern (Lee and Weinblatt, 2001).

Arthritis is a long term condition and progression of the rheumatoid arthritis disease is measured by the disease activity score which has numerous criteria such as number of tender and swollen joints, haemoglobin concentration, morning stiffness duration, CRP and ESR values (Lee and Weinblatt, 2001).

Other inflammatory conditions that could affect cartilage are crystalopathies (gout and pseudogout), ankolysing spondylitis, fibromyalgia, systemic lupus erythemosus, psoriatic arthritis, enteropathic arthritis, reactive arthritis, juvenile arthritis and polymyalgia rheumatica.

Cartilage and Inflammation

Understanding the mechanism of inflammatory resolution would enable permanent treatment of inflammatory conditions. There are numerous mediators that are known to facilitate the acute inflammatory response such as chemokines, cytokines, fibrin, bradykinin, substance P and nitric oxide (Gilroy et al., 2004).

In arthritis, ongoing inflammatory process causes dysregulation of cytokine synthesis which results in destruction of cartilage (Goldring and Berenbaum, 2004). NF-κB pathway is critical in inflammatory process because it not only regulates the expression of cytokines, chemokines and enzymes, but also controls the anti-apoptotic genes (Gilroy et al., 2004).

Increased mechanical loading raises the metabolic activity of chondrocytes and increases production of pro-inflammatory mediators which contributes to the catabolism of chondrocytes (Gosset et al., 2010). This also results in degradation of the matrix. IL-1β, TNF-α and PGE$_2$ are the inflammatory mediators that raise in inflammation.

Current therapeutics that are used to diminish inflammation are NSAIDs which block COX, glucocorticoids that prevent cytokines and biological agents that target specific modulators (Ahmed et al., 2013). Cyclo-oxygenase (COX) enzymes are important for PGE$_2$ formation (Smith et al., 1996) which is a very significant pro-inflammatory product in arthritis. COX has a function in catabolisation of prostaglandin and thromboxane A_2 formation from arachidonic acid (Smith et al., 1996). In prostaglandin H_2 (PGH_2), formation catalysed by COX enzymes; this is converted to PGE_2 by prostaglandin E synthase (PGES).

Pro-inflammatory cytokines assist induction of both PGE_2 and PGES (Murakami et al., 2000). PGE_2 and PGD_2 are the major prostaglandins synthesised by chondrocytes. Although PGE_2 has demonstrated anabolic effects at lower concentrations, presence of higher concentrations lead to apoptosis and erosion of the cartilage (DiBattista et al., 1996; Attur et al., 2008).

Increased COX-2 expression leads to increased PGE_2 levels which cause increased chondrocyte apoptosis and osteoarthritis (Goldring and Berenbaum, 2004). PGD_2 also was found to decrease the viability of chondrocytes (Zhu et al., 2010).

TNF-α and IL-1β activates the NF-κB signalling pathway leading to activation of genes responsible from catabolism and pro-inflammatory functions in cellular level (Liu-Bryan and Terkeltaub, 2010). TNF-α is recognised by TNF Receptor Type 1 (TNFR1) throughout the whole body and TNF Receptor Type 2 (TNFR2) locally in the immune system (Hehlglans and Pfeffer, 2005). When TNF-α binds to TNFR1, it activates the death domain. The importance of TNF-α in osteoarthritis formation could be seen from the evidence of raised amount of TNFR1 in chondrocytes isolated from osteoarthritic joints (Westacott et al., 1994).

In the resolving phase of acute inflammatory process, it is found that there is peak in IL-10 and tissue growth factor β1 (TGF-β1) expression (Gilroy et al., 2004). Fibroblast growth factor 2 (FGF-2) and TGF β1 improve cell proliferation and protect the ability of cells to redifferentiate (Blitterswijk et al., 2005). TGF-β stimulates chondrocyte proliferation and repairing because application of TGFβ increases the gene expression of aggrecan and collagen (Roberts, 1999; Critchlow et al., 1995; Umlauf et al., 2010).

FGFs cause increased cell proliferation and damaged cartilage repair in vitro (Ellman et al., 2008); however, there are several contradictory in vitro studies to this finding (Moore et al., 2005; Umlauf et al., 2010).

Many cellular molecules have been found to have anti-inflammatory effects. Annexin 1 (Hannon et al., 2003), melanocortin (Scholzen et al., 2003) and galectin (La et al., 2003) are found to be able to decrease inflammation in cartilage.

Annexin 1 is suggested to mediate the anti-inflammatory corticosteroid effects (Roviezzo et al., 2002) since the pro-inflammatory cytokines are found to enhance the function of Annexin 1 and animal studies have proven the anti-inflammatory characteristics of Annexin 1 (Perretti et al., 1993). Annexin 1 functions in cell proliferation and phagocytosis as well as mediating the action of glucocorticoids in an inflammatory condition (Roviezzo et al., 2002).

Melanocortin is also important for inflammation process in the body as melanocortin peptides also have anti-inflammatory properties. α-melanocytic stimulating hormone (α-MSH) is found to facilitate the anti-inflammatory process (Catania et al., 2004). Melanocortin receptor 1 and melanocortin receptor 3 are the primary anti-inflammatory melanocortin receptors. MC 1 mediates pro-inflammatory cytokines and MMPs (Grassel et al., 2009). MC 2, on the other hand, causes a decrease in pro-inflammatory and increase in anti-inflammatory mediators (Lam et al., 2005).

α-MSH is detected in very low concentrations in osteoarthritis and rheumatoid arthritis synovial fluid but higher than the plasma concentration meaning that there is local production in inflammation (Catania et al., 1999). α-MSH supresses production of pro-inflammatory cytokines through preventing activation of NF-kB (Manna and Aggarwal, 1998) as well as activating anti-inflammatory cytokines like IL-10 (Bhardwaj et al., 1996).

Further research is required for melanocortin because this is one of the factors that is promising to offer a solution to resolving inflammation. Galectines, inhibitors of chronic inflammation have been under interest as well (Norling et al., 2009). IL-6 is also taught to be important in inflammation since it could facilitate in both inflammatory and anti-inflammatory processes.

Apart from obesity applying increased loading to cartilage, adipokines could affect inflammation as well (Pottie et al., 2006); and what is more, locally produced adipokines could cause destruction. Adiponectin on the other hand, has a protective role against osteoarthritis (Conde et al., 2011).

IL-8 is a chemokine that activates neutrophils and facilitates angiogenesis (Belperio et al., 2000). This chemokine also has a function in mediating inflammation. Synthesis of IL-8 by chondrocytes increases in arthritis (Recklies and Golds, 1992).

Loading on cartilage in physiological limits prevents cartilage degradation by inhibiting activation of NF-κB pathway (Dossumbekova et al., 2007). IL-6 is also a potent pleiotropic cytokine found in chondrocytes (Wong et al., 2010) which facilitates anti-inflammatory as well as pro-inflammatory functions (Goldring, 2000). IL-10 anti-inflammatory cytokine levels are high in chondrocytes of osteoarthritic joints. It supresses TNF-α, IL-1β and IL-6 expression in cartilage tissue. IL-10 also has a function in induction of heme oxygenase 1 (HO-1) which is a protective agent from tissue injury as it removes the free nerve and reduces cellular stress as well as protecting the tissue from cellular damage.

In osteoarthritis, chondrocyte apoptosis is found to be associated with initiation and development of the disease (Kim et al., 2000). Apoptosis could be initiated intracellularly or extracellularly. Internal initiation of apoptosis could take place by mutation or damage of DNA and the external initiation could be done by cytokines. For example, TNFR1 activation by TNF-α initiates apoptosis.

In the cartilage tissue affected by arthritis, increased activity is present through NF-κB pathway. IL-1β and TNF-α can activate catabolic pathways; and, induce iNOS, MMPs, COX-2 and aggreanase (Abramson and Attur, 2009). Caspase proteinases also facilitate apoptosis. Caspase proteinases, especially caspase 3 and caspase 8, is raised in cartilage affected by osteoarthritis (Robertson et al., 2006). Capsase 8 has a function in initiation step of apoptosis whereas capsase 3 has a function in carrying out the process of apoptosis (Lee et al., 2002).

Proteinases also have an important function in healthy cartilage tissue maintenance. They facilitate the equilibrium between cartilage formation and degradation by either degrading extracellular matrix of cartilage and causing joint deformity or degrading the inhibitors and preventing osteoarthritis (Kevorkian et al., 2004).

Matrix metalloproteinases (MMPs) facilitate various processes such as blood coagulation or collagen synthesis (Dickinson, 2002). Expression of MMPs is controlled by growth factors and cytokines. MMP-1 and MMP-3 are the main collagenase matrix proteinases expressed by cartilage in proliferation and osteoarthritis although MMP-1, MMP-8 and MMP-13 are all abundant in cartilage affected from osteoarthritis. These proteinases are able to degrade the interstitial collagen and cause dysfunction (Kevorkian et al., 2004; Martel-Pelletier et al., 2000). Also, IL-1β and TNF-α escalates MMP-1, 3 and 13 expression as well as decreasing type 2 collagen (Bau et al., 2002). MMP-3 is increased in osteoarthritic cartilage (Glasson, 2007) and MMP-3 is an enzyme that has an important function in activation of rest of the MMPs (Tetlow et al., 2001).

Type of compression applied on cartilage is significant and could create proliferative or degenerative changes in signalling pathways. Chondrocytes are mechanosensitive and they alter differently to various forces applied by changing rate of ECM synthesis and proliferation on degradation (Knight et al., 2002) by modification in the signalling pathways.

Dynamic compression has a stimulatory effect (Buschmann et al., 1995). However, dynamic compression receives various responses from different zones of cartilage. The superficial zone cells demonstrate an improvement in cell proliferation by 1 Hertz loading through down-regulation of nitric oxide (Murrell, 1995) whereas deep zone cells increase the synthesis of proteoglycan (Lee et al., 1998).

Although cell proliferation is not dependent on frequency of force application, it is vital for proteoglycan synthesis (Lee and Bader, 1997). TGF-β, in dynamic compression, improves proteoglycan synthesis as well as cell proliferation. α5β1 is the main mechanical stimulus signalling pathway receptor and loading within normal forces in an abnormal physiological condition or abnormal loading within a normal physiology leads to damage of cartilage (Chowdhury, 2001).

α5β1 integrin competitive ligands block the response to loading leading to prevention of cell proliferation and proteoglycan synthesis (Chowdhury et al., 2004). IL-1β increases nitric oxide release which inhibits anabolic pathways (Chowdhury et al., 2001).

Dynamic compression, also, inhibits COX-2 and inducible nitric oxide synthase (iNOS) expression as well as nitric oxide and PGE$_2$ release (Chowdhury et al., 2001). This is important because in osteoarthritis, there is an increase in iNOS which results in increased amounts of nitric oxide production (Martel-Pelletier and Pelletier, 2010).

Problems Encountered in Cartilage Regeneration

One of the most challenging problems in cartilage regeneration is that the growth of chondrocytes in vitro into a monolayer culture causes dedifferentiation, loss of ability to redifferentiate and loss of phenotype (Benya et al., 1982); therefore, there is search for a three dimensional system that could economically provide an optimum environment for chondrocyte growth without loss of morphology.

Three dimensional scaffolding is also important to stimulate extracellular matrix synthesis and preserve the chondrocyte phenotype (Blitterswijk et al., 2005). However, the main problem of three dimensional models is that they do not provide an efficient nutrient and waste product transport to deep zones of cartilage and chondrocytes in the deep region have reduced viability (Heywood, 2005). This situation results in non-homogenous distribution of the chondrocyte density (Choudhury, 2011).

Three dimensional agarose or alginate constructs have been successful in preserving the cell phenotype and permitting spherical chondrocyte formation which preserves the extracellular matrix synthesis and protection of weight-bearing properties. However, matrix interactions are not preserved in these constructs and alterations in mechanosignalling take place (Lee and Bader, 1995; Chowdhury, 2011).

These models are the most frequently used constructs in biomedical research. Apart from three-dimensional scaffolding, matrix requirements for chondrocyte regeneration are porosity to allow cell migration, matrix production as well as nutrient and waste transport; biodegradability and biocompatibility to allow cartilage formation and remodelling; and, elasticity to stand for load application (Freed et al., 1994). Three dimensional model; despite all the advantages, is still not able to imitate the loading experienced in the real life (Chowdhury et al., 2001).

Tissue regeneration field also has an interest in cartilage proliferation. Bioreactors aiming to monitor the optimum medium for chondrocyte proliferation by equal distribution of nutrient delivery and waste removal, including the core region, are trying to be achieved (Heywood, 2005).

Available Cartilage Repair Methods

In order to achieve cartilage repair, healing and regeneration are aimed via either repair of the cartilage internally or by initiation of regeneration by new cells with potential to regenerate.

Currently, a treatment achieving complete repair of damaged chondrocytes locally is not available. Treatments aim to reduce inflammation in long term management, provide pain and symptom relief as well as improving the mobility of the patient by restoring the joint function.

NSAIDs, glucocorticoids and biologicals and DMARDs are the main approaches in medical treatment of arthritis. NSAIDs possess numerous functions such as anti-pyretic effects and pain relief as well as anti-inflammatory effects; however, these medications only provide symptomatic relief to patients and do not alter the disease pathogenesis.

NSAIDs inhibit COX, inhibiting prostaglandin synthesis. The most common side effect of this process is gastrointestinal manifestations. Traditional NSAIDs are non-selective COX inhibitors. However, it is known that COX-2 is elevated in inflammation while COX-1 levels do not change in inflammation. COX-1 has an important function in gastrointestinal system where by production of prostaglandin, it decreases secretion of the gastric acid. This is the main reason for experienced side effects of NSAIDs (Lazzaroni and Bianchi Porro, 2004).

26

This major side effect led to a research for selective COX-2 inhibitors which will dismiss the unwanted side effects due to COX-1 inhibition and only inhibit the function of COX-2. Celecoxib and Rofecoxib, the selective COX-2 inhibitors, also demonstrated a very crucial side effect which was very significant increase in myocardial infarction rate (Mukherjee et al., 2001). The reason for this was found as the disturbance of the balance between Thromboxane A_2 and PGI_2 production leading to decrease of PGI_2 which is a platelet aggregation inhibitor; and, consequent increase in cardiovascular risk due to this (Cannon et al., 2006). Because of this side effect, refecoxib was withdrawn from the market.

Glucocorticoids are steroid hormones that have a function in regulation of inflammation. They are known to inhibit COX-2 leading to inhibition of prostaglandin production. Glucocorticoids prevent vasodilation which is the preliminary stage of inflammation. Also, they prevent increase of vessel permeability to reduce the amount of exudate formed (Perretti and Ahluwalia, 2000).

Glucocorticoids have side effects of immunodeficiency and cushingoid symptoms such as thinning of skin, easy bruising, abnormal fat distribution leading to accumulation of fat tissue in central abdominal region and osteoporosis leading to bone fractures. These side effects and risk of having Cushing's syndrome create a difficulty for use of glucocorticoids in long term.

Biologicals are another choice of treatment in arthritis. The aim of these medications is the inhibition of TNF-α. TNF-α is targeted by monoclonal antibodies and this is used in treatment of various arthritis types including rheumatoid arthritis. Etanercept, infliximab and adalimumab are the biologicals currently used. These medications have shown to create a significant improvement in chronic arthritis; however, body immune system becomes significantly weaker with these medications and the immune system becomes more susceptible to acquiring opportunistic infections. Moreover, anaemia, thrombocytopenia and lymphoma could be caused by biologicals (Dixon et al., 2010; Lee et al., 2007). Therefore, careful monitoring, regular vaccinations and periodical blood tests must be provided to patients.

Healing of hyaline cartilage is restricted (Mankin, 1974; Dowthwaite et al., 2004). Current cartilage repair alternatives are debridement, marrow stimulation, autologous osteochondral transplantation (OATS), autologous chondrocyte implantation (ACI) and allogenic osteochondral transplantation.

Debridement provides temporary pain relief by narrowing the injured cartilage; however, this method does not repair the cartilage, it only provides symptomatic relief. Marrow stimulation, by drilling through cartilage, causes bleeding in the subchondral region to stimulate the bone marrow and initiate repair with fibrous tissue. OATS, also called mosaicplasty, targets to replace the injured cartilage with numerous osteochondral autograft transfers from non-weight bearing areas.

ACI involves taking a cartilage biopsy, expansion of chondrocytes externally, transplantation of newly grown chondrocytes to site of defect and replacement of chondrocytes in the defect site by periosteal grafting. ACI has been the most prevalent application of regenerative medicine (Hausser and Fussenger, 2007).

Allogenic transplantation from cadaveric donor is also a successful method in terms of immunocompatibility due to immunosuppressed nature of cartilage; however, application is limited because of donor unavailability (Zimmer, 2009).

Although these methods are available, adequate data on their short and long term success is not available; and, joint replacement is still the most commonly preferred surgical management technique. Osteotomy, creating a non-functioning joint by merging bones is usually used as a palliative surgical management in extremely painful cases of osteoarthritis.

Impact of Cartilage Damage on Public Health

Osteoarthritis is the most commonly encountered arthritis type and rheumatoid arthritis is the most common inflammatory joint disorder in the UK. Inflammatory and degenerative joint conditions are very common in the developed world. 250 million people on the world suffers from osteoarthritis of knee joint (Vos et al., 2010) and 43 million people are severely disabled due to osteoarthritis (WHO, 2008).

In Europe, almost a quarter of adult population have reported to have arthritis (Health in EU, 2007). World Health Organisation have announced that osteoarthritis is the third greatest cause of disability in global burden (Global Burden of Disease, 2004).

Rheumatoid arthritis affects 1% of the adult population in the developed world and results in approximately 50.000 deaths every year (Scott et al., 2010; Lozano et al., 2012). One in every two elderly above the age of 80 experiences painful osteoarthritis of knees (Peat et al., 2008).

Arthritis of joints results in pain and loss of joint function in patients. Both osteoarthritis and rheumatoid arthritis are long term conditions and a cumulatively growing population is experiencing these conditions every year. In the UK, there are approximately 20.000 new rheumatoid arthritis cases every year. Osteoarthritis incidence also have increased by 30% in the last 10 years (Lawrence et al., 1998; Lawrence et al., 2008). Almost 9 million people living in the UK are receiving treatment for arthritis and 4.7 million of this is knee joint (Arthritis UK, 2009). 6 million painful knee and 2.2 million painful hip osteoarthritis is reported in the UK (Odding et al., 1998; Lanyon et al., 2003).

Involvement of disability and long term treatment create a burden on the society and healthcare system as well as the individual patients. Loss of joint function leads to inability of patients to work and perform advanced daily living activities; resulting in physical problems as well as psychological stress. This also places a burden on the society by means of reduced workforce and increased caring need. Arthritis is the most common cause of obtaining disability living allowance in the UK (Arthritis UK, 2014).

Long term and expensive treatment of these conditions place a financial burden and increased workload on National Health System. Musculoskeletal disorders account for 38% of all occupational health diseases in the European Union (Woolf et al., 2012). This demonstrates a great reduction in workforce as well as increase in caring needs.

In the UK, 58.952 primary hip and 62.150 primary knee replacements took place in 2006 (Arthro Scotland, 2008). The cost of one hip replacement to NHS is £7.350 on average (R de Vertevil et al., 2008). Overall, musculoskeletal conditions cost £5.7 billion on average to NHS every year (Health and Safety Executive, 2008).

In the UK, National Institute for Clinical Excellence (NICE) guidelines have been created to standardise the management and treatment of both osteoarthritis and rheumatoid arthritis.

According to guidelines, osteoarthritis diagnosis is set to patients with: age over 45 (except early onset), activity related joint pain and presence or absence of morning stiffness lasting over 30 minutes. Clinical diagnosis is made by x-ray (Osteoarthritis Overview, 2014). Rheumatoid arthritis is diagnosed by blood test that checks presence of rheumatoid factor followed by anti-cyclic citrullinated peptide antibodies (Managing RA, 2014).

For treatment of both conditions, a stepwise management plan has been created starting with lifestyle modifications followed by medications and finally surgery.

Currently, all treatment modalities aim to temporarily manage these conditions rather than to provide a complete treatment. Research for understanding the inflammatory process in cartilage, functioning of chondrocytes and anti-inflammatory modulators would create a pathway for providing a permanent treatment to the condition and decrease the level of disability within population as well as the long term treatment costs. Until then, public health promotion campaigns are aiming to prevent occurrence of arthritis.

Primary prevention is regular exercise, achieving body weight within normal limits and eating a balanced diet to prevent cartilage damage. Secondary prevention is early intervention to prevent arthritis from progressing.

Media is an important factor for public health promotion and advertisement. Currently, Arthritis UK is the main charity for promoting primary and secondary prevention of arthritic conditions as well as creating funds and support for research to find a cure for these conditions.

World Health Organisation and United Nations, by bone and joint decade, are aiming to reduce the disease burden and cost of musculoskeletal conditions through health promotion and are trying to make musculoskeletal conditions a health priority in health policies of governments.

Conclusion

Degenerative and inflammatory joint conditions are very common amongst population and permanent treatment for chondrocyte repair is still unavailable. Achieving cartilage repair would significantly contribute to an increased quality of life in arthritis patients.

All current management modalities aim to decrease the pain and inflammation as well as preventing progression. Repairing or regenerating damaged chondrocytes is very challenging due to structure of cartilage; however, supressing the inflammation that primarily cause the damage would inhibit degenerative joint diseases.

Although many components, modulators and pathways of the inflammation process is identified, further research with a multidisciplinary approach is still needed in order to find a permanent solution. In the future, development of therapies that could mimic anti-inflammatory mediator actions and prevent chondrocyte damage could achieve resolution of the inflammatory joint diseases.

Acknowledgements

I would like to express my thankfulness to my supervisor Professor Mauro Perretti and Magdalena Kaneva for supporting me in every step of this project. Also, I would like to thank my medical school Barts and the London School of Medicine and Dentistry for giving me every opportunity to continue my research on bone and cartilage regeneration and supporting me in every decision I have made.

I believe my family is my greatest luck and most important thing I have in this life. I would like to thank my family for their love, care and support.

References

Abramson SB, Attur M (2009) Developments in the scientific understanding of osteoarthritis. *Arthritis Res Ther,* 11(3):227,4206.

Ahmed TJ, Montero-Melendez T, Perretti M, Pitzalis C (2013) Curbing inflammation through endogenous pathways: Focus on melanocortin peptides, *International Journal of Inflammation,* 2013:985815.

Arroll B, Goodyear-Smith F (2004) Corticosteroid injections for osteoarthritis of the knee: meta-analysis. *BMJ,* 328 (7444):869.

Arthritis Research UK (2009) National Primary Care Centre, Keele University, Musculoskeletal Matters, Online Resource, Accessible at:http://www.arthritisresearchuk.org/arthritis-information/data-and-statistics/osteoarthritis.aspx#sthash.93NqEoZ8.dpuf, [Date accessed: 30-5-2014].

Arthritis UK (2014) Booklet of Key Facts.

Arthro Scot (2014) Arthritis Scotland, Online Resource, Accessible at: http://www.arthro.scot.nhs.uk/New_Developments/Main.html [Date accessed: 29-2014].

Attur M, Al-Mussawir HE, Patel J, Kitay A, Dave M, Palmer G, Pillinger MH, Abramson SB (2008) Prostaglandin E2 exerts catabolic effects in osteoarthritis cartilage: evidence for signalling via the EP4 receptor. *J Immunol,* 181:5082-8.

Bader DL, Salter DM, Chowdhury TT (2011) Biomechanical Influence of Cartilage Homeostasis in Health and Disease, *Arthritis,* 979032.

Bau B, Gebhard PM, Haag J, Knorr T, Bartnik E, Aigner T (2002) Relative messenger RNA expression profiling of collagenases and aggrecanases in human articular chondrocytes in vivo and in vitro. *Arthritis Rheum,* 46:2648-57.

Belperio JA, Keane MP, Arenberg DA, Addison CL, Ehlert JE, Burdic MD, Strieter RM (2000) CXC chemokines in angiogenesis. *J Leukoc Biol,* 68:1-8.

Benya PD, Shaffer JD (1982) Dedifferentiated chondrocytes reexpress the differentiated collagen phenotype when cultured in agarose gels, *Cell,* 30(1):215-24.

Bhardwaj RS, Schwarz A, Becher E, Mahnke K, Aragane Y, Schwarz T, Luger TA (1996) Pro-opiomelanocortin-derived peptides induce IL-10 production in human monocytes. *J Immunol,* 156:2517-21.

Biswas S, Sharma S, Saroha A, Bhakuni DS, Malhotra R, Zahur M, Oellerich M, Das HR, Asif AR (2013) Identification of Novel Autoantigen in the Synovial Fluid of Rheumatoid Arthritis Patients Using an Immunoproteomics Approach. *PLoS ONE,* 8(2), e56246.

Blitterswijk CV et al. (2005) Tissue Engineering, 537-539, Elsevier.

Buckwalter JA and Mankin HJ (1998) Articular cartilage: degeneration and osteoarthritis, repair, regeneration, and transplantation. *Instr Course Lect,* 47:487-504.

Buschmann MD, Kim YJ, Wong M, Frank E, Hunziker EB, Grodzinsky AJ (1995) Stimulation of Aggrecan Synthesis in Cartilage Explants by Cyclic Loading Is Localized to Regions of High Interstitial Fluid Flow, *Cell Sci,* 108:1497-508.

Cannon CP, Curtis SP, Fitzgerald GA, Krum H, Kaur A, Bolognese JA, Reicin AS, Bombardier C, Weinblatt ME, Van Der Heijde D, Erdmann E, Laine L (2006) Cardiovascular outcomes with etoricoxib and diclofenac in patients with osteoarthritis and rheumatoid arthritis in the Multinational Etoricoxib and Diclofenac Arthritis Long-term (MEDAL) programme: a randomised comparison. *Lancet,* 368:1771-81.

Catania A, Delgado R, Airaghi L, Cutuli M, Garofalo L, Carlin A, Demitri MT, Lipton JM (1999) Alpha-MSH in systemic inflammation. Central and peripheral actions. *Ann N Y Acad Sci,* 885:183-7.

Catania A, Gatti S, Colombo G, Lipton JM (2004) Targeting melanocortin receptors as a novel strategy to control inflammation. *Pharmacol Rev,* 56:1-29.

Chowdhury T (2011) Cartilage and Bioreactors Lectures, Tissue Engineering and Regenerative Medicine, Queen Mary University of London.

Chowdhury T, Bader DL, Lee DA (2001) Dynamic compression inhibits the synthesis of Nitric Oxide and PGE_2 by IL-1β-Stimulated Chondrocytes Cultured in Agarose Constructs, *Biochemical and Biophysical Research Communications*, 285, 1168-74.

Chowdhury T, Salter DM, Bader DL, Lee DA (2004) Integrin-mediated mechanoconstruction processes in TGFβ-stimulated monolayer-expanded chondrocytes, *BBRC*, 318:873-881.

Cohen NP, Foster RJ, Mow MC (1998) Composition and dynamics of articular cartilage: structure, function, and maintaining, *J Orthop Sports Phys Ther,* 28(4)203-15.

Colledge NR, Walker BR, Ralston S, Davidson S (2010) Davidson's principles and practice of medicine. Edinburgh: Churchill Livingstone/Elsevier.

Conde J, Gomez R, Bianco G, Scotece M, Lear P, Dieguez C, Gomez-Reino J, Lago F, Gualillo O (2011) Expanding the adipokine network in cartilage: identification and regulation of novel factors in human and murine chondrocytes. *Ann Rheum Dis.,* 70:551–9.

Critchlow MA, Bland YS, Ashhurst DE (1995) The effect of exogenous transforming growth factor-beta 2 on healing fractures in the rabbit. *Bone,* 16(5):521–527.

de Verteuil R, Imamura , Zhu S, Glazener C, Fraser C, Munro N, Hutchison J, Grant A, Coyle D, Coyle K, Vale L (2008) A systematic review of the clinical effectiveness and cost-effectiveness and economic modelling of minimal incision total hip replacement approaches in the management of arthritic disease of the hip. *Health Technol Assess,* 12(26):1-244.

Dibattista JA, Dore S, Morin N, Abribat T (1996) Prostaglandin E2 up-regulates insulin-like growth factor binding protein-3 expression and synthesis in human articular chondrocytes by a c-AMP-independent pathway: role of calcium and protein kinase A and C. *J Cell Biochem,* 63:320-33.

Dickinson DP (2002) Cysteine peptidases of mammals: their biological roles and potential effects in the oral cavity and other tissues in health and disease. *Crit Rev Oral Biol Med,* 1:238-75.

Dixon WG, Hyrich KL, Watson KD, Lunt M, Galloway J, Ustianowski A, Symmons DP (2010) Drug-specific risk of tuberculosis in patients with rheumatoid arthritis treated with anti-TNF therapy: results from the British Society for Rheumatology Biologics Register. *Ann Rheum Dis,* 69:522-8.

Dossumbekova A, Anghelina M, Madhavan S, He L, Quan N, Knobloch T, Agarwal S (2007) Biomechanical signals inhibit IKK activity to attenuate NF-kappa B transcription activity in inflamed chondrocytes. *Arthritis Rheum,* 56:3284-96.

Dowthwaite GP, Bishop JC, Redman SN, Khan IM, Rooney P, Evans DJR, Haughton L, Bayram Z, Boyer S, Thomson B, Wolfe MS, Archer CW (2004) The surface of articular cartilage contains a progenitor cell population. *J Cell Sci,* 117(6):889-97.

Ellman MB, An HS, Muddasani P, Im HJ (2008) Biological impact of the fibroblast growth factor family on articular cartilage and intervertebral disc homeostasis. *Gene,* 420:82-9.

Freed LE, Vunak G, Biron RJ, Eagles DB, Lesnoy DC, Barlow SK, Langer R (1994) Biodegradable polymer scaffolds for tissue engineering, *Biotechnology (NY),* 12:689-693.

Gibson T, Davis WB, Curran RC (1958) The long term survival of cartilage omografts in man. *Br J Plast Surg,* 11:177-87.

Gilroy DW, Lawrence T, Perretti M, Rossi AG (2004) Inflammatory resolution: new opportunities for drug discovery. *Nat. Rev. Drug. Discov,* 3:401-16.

Glasson SS (2007) In vivo osteoarthritis target validation utilizing genetically-modified mice. *Curr Drug Targets,* 8(2):367–76.

Global Burden of Disease (2004) Table 9: Estimated prevalence of moderate and severe disability (millions) for leading disabling conditions by age, for high-income and low- and middle-income countries, 2004. Geneva: World Health Organization, 35.

Goldring MB (2000) Osteoarthritis and cartilage: the role of cytokines. *Curr Rheumatol Rep,* 2:459-65.

Goldring MB, Berenbaum F (2004) The regulation of chondrocyte function by proinflammatory mediators: prostaglandins and nitric oxide. *Clin Orthop Relat Res*:37-46.

Gosset M, Pigenet A, Salvat C, Berenbaum F, Jacques C (2010) Inhibition of matrix metalloproteinase-3 and -13 synthesis induced by IL-1beta in chondrocytes from mice lacking microsomal prostaglandin E synthase-1. *J Immunol,* 185:6244-52.

Grassel S, Opolka A, Anders S, Straub RH, Grifka J, Luger TA, Bohm M (2009) The melanocortin system in articular chondrocytes: melanocortin receptors, pro-opiomelanocortin, precursor proteases, and a regulatory effect of alpha-melanocyte-stimulating hormone on proinflammatory cytokines and extracellular matrix components. *Arthritis Rheum,* 60:3017-27.

Grodzinsky AJ, Schunke M (2004) Influence of tissue maturation and antioxidants on the apoptotic response of articular cartilage after injurious compression. *Arthritis Rheum,* 50:123-30.

Gross AE, Sasha N, Aubin P (2008) Fresh osteochondral allografts for posttraumatic knee defects: Long-term followup. *Clin Orthop Relat Res,* 466:1863-1870.

Hall AG (1998) Physiology of Cartilage. *Saunders.*

Hannon R, Croxtall JD, Getting SJ, Roviezzo F, Yona S, Paul-Clark MJ, Gavins FN, Perretti M, Morris JF, Buckingham JC, Flower RJ (2003) Aberrant inflammation and resistance to glucocorticoids in annexin 1-/- mouse. *Faseb J,* 17:253-5.

Hausser H, Fussenegger M (2007) Tissue Engineering, 237-249 Second Edition, Humana Press.

Health and Safety Executive (2008) Musculoskeletal disorders – Why tackle them?, Online resource, Accessed at: http://www.hse.gov.uk/healthservices/msd/whytackle.htm [Date accessed: 7-5-2014].

Health in the European Union (2007) Special Eurobarometer 272e. European Commission, Online Research, Accessed at: http://ec.europa.eu/health/ph_ publication/eb_health_en.pdf. Online resource, Accessed at: http://www.arthritisresearchuk.org/health-professionals-and-students/reports/topical-reviews/topical-reviews-summer-2012.aspx#sthash.vlx7Uvtq.dpuf, [Date accessed: 7-5-12].

Hehlgans T, Pfeffer K (2005) The intriguing biology of the tumour necrosis factor/tumour necrosis factor receptor superfamily: players, rules and the games. *Immunology,* 115:1-20.

Heywood HK Nalesso G, Lee DA, Oomens CW, Bader DL (2005) Nutrient utilization by bovine articular chondrocytes: a combined experimental and theoretical approach, *J. Biomech. Eng*, 127(5):758.

Heywood HK, Bader DL, Lee DA (2006) Rate of oxygen consumption by isolated articular chondrocytes is sensitive to medium glucose concentration, *Journal of Cellular Physiology,* 206(2):402–10.

Hunter W (1743) Of the structure and diseases of articulating cartilages. *Phil Trans,* 42:514–21. [Clin Ortop Relat Res (1995) 317:3-6].

Husing B, Senker J, Kirkpatrick CJ (2003), Human Tissue Engineered Products –Today's Markets and Future Prospects, Fraunhofer Institute for Systems and Innovation Research, Karlsruhe, Germany.

Kevorkian L, Young DA, Darrah C, Donell ST, Shepstone L, Porter S, Brockbank SM, Edwards DR, Parker AE, Clark IM (2004) Expression profiling of metalloproteinases and their inhibitors in cartilage. *Arthritis Rheum,* 50:131-41.

Kim HA, Blanco FJ (2007) Cell death and apoptosis in osteoarthritic cartilage. *Curr Drug Targets,* 8:333-45.

Kim HA, Lee YJ, Seong SC, Choe KW, Song YW (2000) Apoptotic chondrocyte death in human osteoarthritis. *J Rheumatol,* 27:455-62.

Knight MM, Van De Breevaart Bravenboer J, Lee DA, van Osch GJ, Weinans H, Bader DL (2002) Cell and nucleus deformation in compressed chondrocyte-alginate constructs: Temporal changes and calculation of cell modulus. *Biochimica et Biophysica Acta,* 1570(1):1-8.

Kuhnel W (2003) Color Atlas of Cytology, Histology and Microscopic Anatomy, 193, Thieme.

Kunisch E, Jansen A, Kojima F, Loffler I, Kapoor M, Kawai S, Rubio I, Crofford LJ, Kinne RW (2009) Prostaglandin E2 differentially modulates proinflammatory/prodestructive effects of TNFalpha on synovial fibroblasts via specific E prostanoid receptors/cAMP. *J Immunol,* 183:1328-36.

La M, Cao TV, Cerchiaro G, Chilton K, Hirabayashi J, Kasai K, Oliani SM, Chernajovsky Y, Perretti M (2003) A Novel biological activity for galectin-1: inhibition of leukocyte-endothelial cell interactions in experimental inflammation. *Am J Pathol,* 163:1505-15.

Lam CW, Getting SJ, Perretti M (2005) In vitro and in vivo induction of heme oxygenase 1 in mouse macrophages following melanocortin receptor activation. *J Immunol,* 174:2297-304.

Lanyon P, Muir K, Doherty S, Doherty M (2003) Age and sex differences in hip joint space among asymptomatic subjects without structural change: implications for epidemiologic studies. Arthritis Rheum, 48(4):1041-6.

Lawrence RC, Felson DT, Helmick CG, Arnold LM, Choi H, Deyo RA, Gabriel S, Hirsch R, Hochberg MC, Hunder GG, Jordan JM, Katz JN, Kremers HM, Wolfe F (2008) Estimates of the prevalence of arthritis and other rheumatic conditions in the United States. *Arthritis Rheum,* 58:26-35.

Lawrence RC, Helmick CG, Arnett FC, Deyo RA, Felson DT, Giannini EH, Heyse SP, Hirsch R, Hochberg MC, Hunder GG, Liang MH, Pillemer SR, Steen VD, Wolfe F (1998) Estimates of the prevalence of arthritis and selected musculoskeletal disorders in the United States. *Arthritis Rheum,* 41(5):778–799.

Lazzaroni M, Bianchi Porro G (2004) Gastrointestinal side-effects of traditional non-steroidal anti-inflammatory drugs and new formulations. *Aliment Pharmacol Ther,* 20(2):48-58.

Lee DA, Bader DL (1995) The development and characterization of an in vitro system to study strain induced cell deformation in isolated chondrocytes. *In Vitro Cell Dev Biol Anim,* 31(11):828-35.

Lee DA, Bader DL (1997) Compressive strains at physiological frequencies influence the metabolism of chondrocytes seeded in agarose. *J Orthop Res,* 15:181–8.

Lee DA, Noguchi T, Knight MM, O'Donnell L, Bentley G, Bader DL (1998) Response of chondrocyte subpopulations cultured within unloaded and loaded agarose, *J. Orth. Res.* 16(6):726-33.

Lee DM, Weinblatt ME (2001) Rheumatoid arthritis. *Lancet,* 358_(9285):903-11.

Lee TJ, Jang J, Kang S, Jin M, Shin H, Kim DW, Kim BS (2013) Enhancement of osteogenic and chondrogenic differentiation of human embryonic stem cells by mesodermal lineage induction with BMP-4 and FGF2 treatment. *Biochemical and Biophysical Research Communications,* 430(2):793-7.

Lee TS, Chau LY (2002) Heme oxygenase-1 mediates the anti-inflammatory effect of interleukin-10 in mice. *Nat Med,* 8:240-6.

Lee, HH, Song IH, Friedrich M, Gauliard A, Detert J, Rowert J, Audring H, Kary S, Burmester GR, Sterry W, Worm M (2007) Cutaneous side-effects in patients with rheumatic diseases during application of tumour necrosis factor-alpha antagonists. *Br J Dermatol,* 156:486-91.

Liu-Bryan R, Terkeltaub R (2010) Chondrocyte innate immune myeloid differentiation factor 88-dependent signaling drives procatabolic effects of the endogenous Toll-like receptor 2/Toll-like receptor 4 ligands low molecular weight hyaluronan and high mobility group box chromosomal protein 1 in mice. *Arthritis Rheum,* 62:2004-12.

Lozano R, Naghavi M, Foreman K, Lim S, Shibuya K, Aboyans V, Abraham J, Adair T et al. (2012) Global and regional mortality from 235 causes of death for 20 age groups in 1990 and 2010: a systematic analysis for the Global Burden of Disease Study 2010. *Lancet,* 380(9859):2095–128.

Managing RA (2014) NICE, Online Resource, Accessible at: http://pathways.nice.org.uk/pathways/rheumatoid-arthritis/managing-rheumatoid-arthritis, [Date accessed: 29-5-2014].

Mankin HJ (1974) Reaction of articular-cartilage to injury and osteoarthritis. *N Engl J Med*, 291(24):1285-92.

Manna SK, Aggarwal BB (1998) A-melanocyte stimulating hormone inhibits the nuclear transcription factor NF-kB activation induced by various inflammatory agents, *J of Immunol*, 161(6):2873-80.

Marieb EN, Hoehn K (2009) Human Anatomy and Physiology, 131-133, International Edition, Benjamin Cummings, Pearson.

Martel-Pelletier J, Pelletier JP (2010) Is osteoarthritis a disease involving only cartilage or other articular tissues?. *Eklem Hastalik Cerrahisi,* 21:2-14.

Martel-Pelletier J, Welsch DJ, Pelletier JP (2001) Metalloproteases and inhibitors in arthritic diseases. *Best Pract Res Clin Rheumatol,* 15:805-29.

Moore EE, Bendele AM, Thompson DL, Littau A, Waggie KS, Reardon B, Ellsworth JL (2005) Fibroblast growth factor-18 stimulates chondrogenesis and cartilage repair in a rat model of injury-induced osteoarthritis. *Osteoarthr Cartil,* 13(7):623-631.

Mow VC, Wang CC (1999) Some bioengineering considerations for tissue engineering of articular cartilage, *Clin Orthop.,* 367:204-223.

Mukherjee D, Nissen SE, Topol EJ (2001) Risk of cardiovascular events associated with selective COX-2 inhibitors. *JAMA,* 286:954-9.

Mulherin D, Fitzgerald O, Bresnihan B (1996) Clinical improvement and radiological deterioration in rheumatoid arthritis: evidence that the pathogenesis of synovial inflammation and articular erosion may differ. *Br J Rheumatol,* 35:1263-68.

Murakami M, Nakatani Y, Kuwata H, Kudo I (2000) Cellular components that functionally interact with signaling phospholipase A(2)s. *Biochim Biophys Acta,* 1988:159-66.

Murrell GA, Lang D, Williams R (1995) Nitric oxide activates metalloprotease enzymes in articular cartilage. Biochem Biophys Res Commun, 206(1):15-21.

Namba RS, Meuli M, Sullivan KM, Le AX, Adzick NS (1998) Spontaneous repair of superficial defects in articular cartilage in a fetal lamb model. *J Bone Joint Surg Am,* 80(1):4-10.

Norling LV, Perretti M, Cooper D (2009) Endogenous galectins and the control of the host inflammatory response. *J Endocrinol,* 201:169-84.

Odding E, Valkenburg HA, Algra D, Vandenouweland FA, Grobbee DE, Hofman A (1998) Associations of radiological osteoarthritis of the hip and knee with locomotor disability in the Rotterdam Study. *Ann Rheum Dis,* 57(4):203-8.

Osteoarthritis Overview (2014) NICE, Online Resource, Accessible at: http://pathways.nice.org.uk/pathways/osteoarthritis#content=view-node%3Anodes-diagnosis, [Date accessed: 29-5-2014].

Osteoarthritis, (2012), NHS Choices, Online Resource, Accessible at: http://www.nhs.uk/conditions/osteoarthritis/Pages/Introduction.aspx, [Date accessed: 30-5-2014].

Palsson BO, Bhatia SN (2004) Tissue Engineering, 244-67.

Peat G, Duncan R, Thomas E (2008) Data from CAS-K study. Personal communication.

Perretti M and Ahluwalia A (2000) The microcirculation and inflammation: site of action for glucocorticoids, *Microcirculation,* 7(3):147-161.

Perretti M, Ahluwalia A, Harris JG, Goulding NJ, Flower RJ (1993) Lipocortin-1 fragments inhibit neutrophil accumulation and neutrophil-dependent edema in the mouse. A qualitative comparison with an anti-CD11b monoclonal antibody. *J Immunol,* 151:4306-14.

Poole CA, Ayad S, Gilbert RT (1992) Chondrons from articular cartilage. V. Immunohistochemical evaluation of type VI collagen organisation in isolated chondrons by light, confocal and electron microscopy. *J Cell Sci,* 103(4):1101-10.

Pottie P, Presle N, Terlain B, Netter P, Mainard D, Berenbaum F (2006) Obesity and osteoarthritis: more complex than predicted. *Ann Rheum Dis,* 65:1403-1405.

Recklies AD, Golds EE (1992) Induction of synthesis and release of interleukin-8 from human articular chondrocytes and cartilage explants. *Arthritis Rheum,* 35:1509-10.

Roberts AB (1999) TGF-beta signaling from receptors to the nucleus. *Microbes Infect,* 1(15):1265-1273.

Robertson CM, Pennock AT, Harwood FL, Pomerleau AC, Allen RT, Amiel D (2006) Characterization of pro-apoptotic and matrix-degradative gene expression following induction of osteoarthritis in mature and aged rabbits. *Osteoarthritis Cartilage:*14, 471-76.

Roviezzo F, Getting SJ, Paul-Clark MJ, Yona S, Gavins FN, Perretti M, Hannon R, Croxtall JD, Buckingham JC, Flower RJ (2002) The annexin-1 knockout mouse: what it tells us about the inflammatory response. *J Physiol Pharmacol,* 53:541-53.

Scholzen T, Luger TA (1997) Evidence for the differential expression of the functional alpha-melanocyte-stimulating hormone receptor MC-1 on human monocytes. *J Immunol,* 158:3378-84.

Scott DL, Wolfe F, Huizinga TW (2010) Rheumatoid arthritis. *Lancet,* 376:9746:1094-108.

Smith CJ, Sun D, Hoegler C, Roth BS, Zhang X, Zhao G, Xu XB, Kobari Y, Pritchard K, Sessa WC, Hintze TH (1996) Reduced gene expression of vascular endothelial NO synthase and cyclooxygenase-1 in heart failure. *Circ Res,* 78:58-64.

Stockwell RA, Meachim G (1979) The chondrocytes. In Freeman MAR, ed. Adult Articular Cartilage. Tunbridge Wells, England, Pitman Medical, 69-144.

Tetlow LC, Adlam DJ, Woolley DE (2001) Matrix metalloproteinase and proinflammatory cytokine production by chondrocytes of human osteoarthritic cartilage—associations with degenerative changes. *Arthritis Rheum,* 44(3):585-594.

Tortora GJ, Derrickson B (2006) Principles of Anatomy and Physiology, 11th Edition, Wiley, 129-130.

Umlauf D, Svetlana F, Pap T, Bertrand J (2010) Cartilage biology, pathology and repair. *Cellular and Molecular Life Sciences*, 67:4197-4211.

Van Venrooij WJ, Pruijn GJ (2008) An important step towards completing the rheumatoid arthritis cycle. *Arthritis Res Ther,* 10:117.

Van Venrooij WJ, Van Beers JJ, Pruijn GJ (2008) Anti-CCP Antibody, a Marker for the Early Detection of Rheumatoid Arthritis. *Ann NY Acad Sci,* 1143:268-85.

Vos T, Flaxman AD, Naghavi M, Lozano R, Michaud C, Ezzati M, Shibuya K, Salomon JA, Abdalla S, Aboyans V, et al. (2012) Years lived with disability (YLDs) for 1160 sequelae of 289 diseases and injuries 1990-2010: a systematic analysis for the Global Burden of Disease Study 2010. *Lancet,* 380(9859):2163–96.

Wayne C (2012) Columbia Univerity Orthopaedics, Online Resource, Accessible at:http://csu-cvmbs.colostate.edu/academics/clinsci/equine-orthopaedic-research-center/orthopaedic-topics/Pages/equine-joints.aspx, [Date accessed: 24-5-2014].

Westacott CI, Atkins RM, Dieppe PA, Elson CJ (1994) Tumor necrosis factor-alpha receptor expression on chondrocytes isolated from human articular cartilage. *J Rheumatol,* 21:1710-5.

Wheeless CR (2011) Wheeless' Textbook of Orthopaedics, Online Resource, Accessible at:http://www.wheelessonline.com/ortho/articular_cartilage, [Date accessed: 30-5-2014].

WHO (2008) Arthritis Research UK WHO Statistics, Online Resource, Accessible at:http://www.arthritisresearchuk.org/health-professionals-and-students/reports/topical-reviews/topical-reviews-summer-2012.aspx#sthash.vlx7Uvtq.dpuf, [Date accessed: 24-5-2014].

Wong M, Ziring D, Korin Y, Desai S, Kim S, Lin J, Gjertson D, Braun J, Reed E, Singh RR (2008) TNFalpha blockade in human diseases: mechanisms and future directions. *Clin Immunol,* 126:121-36.

Wood NC, Dickens E, Symons JA, Duff GW (1992) In situ hybridization of interleukin-1 in CD14-positive cells in rheumatoid arthritis. *Clin Immunol Immunopathol,* 62:295-300.

Woolf AD, Erwin JE, March L (2012) The need to address the burden of musculoskeletal conditions. *Best Pract Res Clin Rheumatol*, 26(2):183-224.

Xia Y, Wikberg JE, Chhajlani V (1995) Expression of melanocortin 1 receptor in periaqueductal gray matter. *Neuroreport,* 6: 2193-6.

Zhu F, Wang P, Kontrogianni-Konstantopoulos A, Konstantopoulos K (2010) Prostaglandin (Pg)D(2) and 15-Deoxy-Delta(12,14)-Pgj(2), But Not Pge(2), Mediate Shear-Induced Chondrocyte Apoptosis Via Protein Kinase A-Dependent Regulation Of Polo-Like Kinases. *Cell Death Differ,* 17:1325-34.

Zimmer Technical Memo (2009) Articular cartilage repair: basic science, Zimmer.

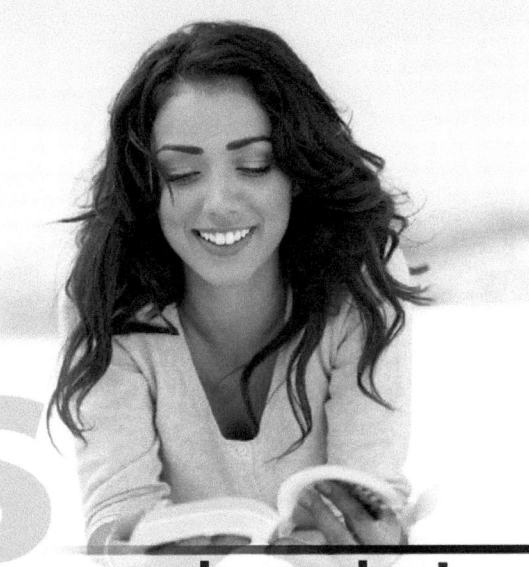
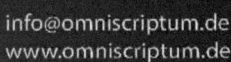
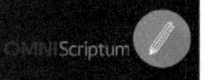

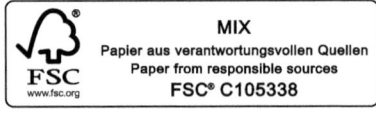